Mariem Nouira
Nesrine Souayeh
Hajer Nouira

Towards the implementation of telemedicine in Tunisia

Mariem Nouira
Nesrine Souayeh
Hajer Nouira

Towards the implementation of telemedicine in Tunisia

Physicians' knowledge and perceptions

ScienciaScripts

Imprint

Cover image: www.ingimage.com

This book is a translation from the original published under ISBN 978-620-6-72106-2.

Publisher:
Sciencia Scripts
is a trademark of
Dodo Books Indian Ocean Ltd. and OmniScriptum S.R.L publishing group

120 High Road, East Finchley, London, N2 9ED, United Kingdom
Str. Armeneasca 28/1, office 1, Chisinau MD-2012, Republic of Moldova, Europe
Printed at: see last page
ISBN: 978-620-8-32978-5

Contents

Resume

Introduction:

The implementation of telemedicine in Tunisia has met with little success and is not very widespread or well known among health professionals, and very few studies have been carried out on the subject.

Methods:

This was a descriptive cross-sectional online study of knowledge, attitudes and practices carried out during October 2022.

Results:

A total of 243 doctors were included. More than half of the doctors (59.3%) had a low level of telemedicine knowledge.

Regarding the evaluation of attitudes, the majority of respondents (89.3%) had an average or high score for the benefits lost. More than three quarters of respondents had a moderate or high score for the degree of lost compatibility of telemedicine with their practice. The majority (93%) had a moderate or high willingness to try telemedicine.

Conclusion:

The positive attitude of Tunisian doctors towards telemedicine and their willingness to try it out in their future practice are encouraging for its widespread implementation in Tunisia.

1 INTRODUCTION

he world today is witnessing rapid advances in audiovisual and digital technologies. The availability of the internet has enabled impressive gains to be made in terms of time and distance. In the light of all this progress, remote medicine is taking place at an increasingly rapid pace (1).

Information and communication technologies (ICTs) are playing an increasingly important and dominant role in the healthcare sector. They represent a multitude of solutions to the various difficulties encountered in practising medicine (2). Telemedicine, one of the most promising means of ICT, is taking on more and more importance in the practice of modern medicine in order to meet the new needs and challenges in the field of health (3).

The World Health Organization defines telemedicine as "The delivery of health care services, where distance is a critical factor, for all health professionals using ICTs to exchange valid information for the diagnosis, treatment and prevention of disease and injury, the evaluation of research and the continuing education of health care providers, with the aim of advancing the health of individuals and their communities" (4).

The term telemedicine was first introduced in Anglo-Saxon medical literature in the 1970s. The history of telemedicine began with the development of epistolary exchanges between doctors (smoke signals, light reflection) to send messages at a distance. With the advent of the Internet came the era of "modern" telemedicine (5).

Telemedicine services were initially reserved for elderly patients with chronic illnesses who were unable to travel to health centres for regular monitoring and control of their illnesses (6,7).

The fields of application of telemedicine were subsequently identified and defined. Telemedicine covers procedures such as teleconsultation, teleexpertise, medical telemonitoring, medical teleassistance, telephonic medical response, etc. (8).

The health crisis caused by the COVID-19 pandemic highlighted the relevance and importance of telemedicine in the medical field. During the pandemic, telemedicine was used more extensively than ever before. Telemedicine thus enabled equitable access to care for all socio-economic categories of patients, improved access to healthcare services for patients who were geographically isolated or had a loss of autonomy, and facilitated coordination between different healthcare providers(9,10).

However, its implementation in Tunisia and other developing countries has met with little success and modest or even limited use for several reasons (11,12). The legal aspects of telemedicine use could be one of the major limitations to its generalisation.

In Tunisia, the legal framework for the practice of telemedicine was obtained following the publication of Presidential Decree no. 318/2022 in April 2022 (13).

However, the practice of the various aspects of telemedicine in Tunisia is not very widespread or well known among health professionals, and very few studies have been carried out on the subject. Doctors are the main and fundamental players in the implementation, practice, maintenance and development of telemedicine. It is therefore essential to take stock of the situation and get a clearer idea of how doctors perceive telemedicine.

This is the background to our study, the main aim of which is to assess the knowledge, attitudes and practices of Tunisian doctors with regard to telemedicine. The secondary objective of our study was to determine the obstacles to its use in medical practice.

2 METHODS

1. Type of study

This is a descriptive cross-sectional online observational study of the Knowledge Attitudes and Practices (KAP) type, which was carried out in October 2022.

2. Study population

Data was collected online using a Google Forms form, which was emailed to a large sample of doctors.

An introductory e-mail explaining the framework of the study and its main objective was sent, stating that the data would be processed with due regard for confidentiality and anonymity. They have been informed that their participation in the study is based purely on their own free will and that they are free to refrain from taking part in the study or to stop replying to the form at any time.

2.1. Inclusion criteria

- Be a qualified Tunisian doctor (general practitioner or specialist) practising in Tunisia during the study period, in the public or private sector, whatever their speciality (general practitioner/family doctor or specialist/university hospital).
- Agreeing to take part in the survey (obtaining consent).

2.2.2.2. Criteria for non-inclusion

Doctors in training (interns/residents) were not included in our study.

1.3. Exclusion criteria

Withdrawal of participation halfway through (Questionnaire not completed to the end).

3. Sampling of the study

The sample for our study was not randomly selected. However, we tried to target a very large number of doctors throughout Tunisia by using an almost exhaustive email list of doctors registered with the Medical Council and the additional email list of all university hospital lecturers belonging to the Faculty of Medicine in Tunis. Our study was carried out online on the basis of voluntary participation and online response to the form sent.

4. Data collection

Data was collected using a structured Google Forms questionnaire distributed online via an email list to a large sample of doctors.

The questionnaire was developed on the basis of a review of the literature on telemedicine. It comprised closed and semi-open items/questions divided into four main parts:

- Basic socio-demographic data (12 questions): age, gender, years of experience, specialism, IT skills, etc.
- Knowledge of telemedicine (5 questions and a score).
- Attitudes towards telemedicine (6 questions and a score).
- Telemedicine practice.

4.1. Knowledge section

The knowledge section was assessed using 12 questions. Participants were asked to answer these questions by selecting "Yes" or "No". Here are some examples of questions that were asked in this section:

"Do you know the benefits of telemedicine?

"Do you know what technologies are used in telemedicine?"

"Do you have any knowledge of the regulations in force concerning the practice of telemedicine?

A knowledge score was assigned to each answer. The "Yes" answer was awarded 1 point and the "No" answer was awarded 0 points.

The total knowledge score could vary from a minimum of 0 to a maximum of 12 in this section.

The level of knowledge was determined using this score, as follows:

- A knowledge score < 6 indicated a low level of knowledge of telemedicine,
- while a score > 6 indicated a good level of telemedicine knowledge.

4.2. Attitudes section

The ATTITUDES section consisted of 4 subsections:

- Perceived benefits.
- Degree of compatibility with practice.
- Ability or willingness to practise telemedicine.
- Threats-complexities-inconveniences.

Participants were asked to indicate their level of agreement or disagreement with various statements about telemedicine.

A 4-point Likert scale was used to measure the attitude score for each section (Strongly agree=4; Agree=3; Don't know (undecided)=2; Disagree =1; Strongly disagree =0). With the exception of the questions on complexity, which were scored inversely (0 = strongly agree and 4 = strongly disagree).

Here are some examples of the questions asked in each section:

- Perceived benefits: "Telemedicine can improve patient access to medical care".

- Degree of compatibility with practice: "I think telemedicine can be integrated effectively into my medical practice".
- Ability or willingness to practice telemedicine: "I am willing to offer remote medical consultations via telemedicine platforms."
- Threats-complexities-inconveniences per^us: "Telemedicine is too complex to implement in my medical practice."

A total score was calculated for each section of the ATTITUDES section. A score of 49% or less was considered low, a score between 50% and 70% as average, and a score of 71% or more as high, thus indicating the participants' level of attitude in each section.

4.3. PRACTICES section

Doctors' practices were evaluated using the following questions:

"Have you ever performed a telemedicine procedure?

"If yes, at what rate?

"If yes, how did you carry out telemedicine procedures?

5. Statistical analysis

For descriptive statistics, categorical variables were expressed in terms of absolute and relative frequencies (percentages), while quantitative variables were expressed as the mean (± standard deviation). The chi-square test was used to compare percentages between the different groups. The Student's t-test was used to compare two means on independent samples. Statistical analysis was performed using SPSS software (version 23.0, IBM Corp). A p value < 0.05 was considered significant.

6. Bibliographic research

We used Zotero for bibliographic management.

The databases consulted during the bibliographic search were : Pubmed, Scopus, Google Scholar and Science direct.

We used the following keywords: telemedicine; information and communication technologies; knowledge; attitudes, practice; doctors; Tunisia.

7. Ethical considerations

All participants were informed of the framework and main objective of the study prior to their participation and were cordially invited to take part on a voluntary basis. All this information was mentioned in the text of the Google Forms form sent by e-mail. They were also informed of their right to refuse to participate or to withdraw from the data collection process at any time. All data collected and analysed was treated anonymously. Data confidentiality was respected during and after data collection. The approval of the Ethics Committee of the Ben Arous Regional Hospital was obtained before the study was carried out, with the approval number 11/2022.

3 RESULTS

I. Socio-professional characteristics

A total of 243 doctors took part in the study. More than half (57.2%) were women, with a sex ratio (F/H) = 1.33. Participants ranged in age from 30 to 72 years. The mean age was 45 ± 9.6 years, with a significant gender difference (48.4 years for men vs. 42.4 years for women, $p<10^{-3}$) (Figure 1).

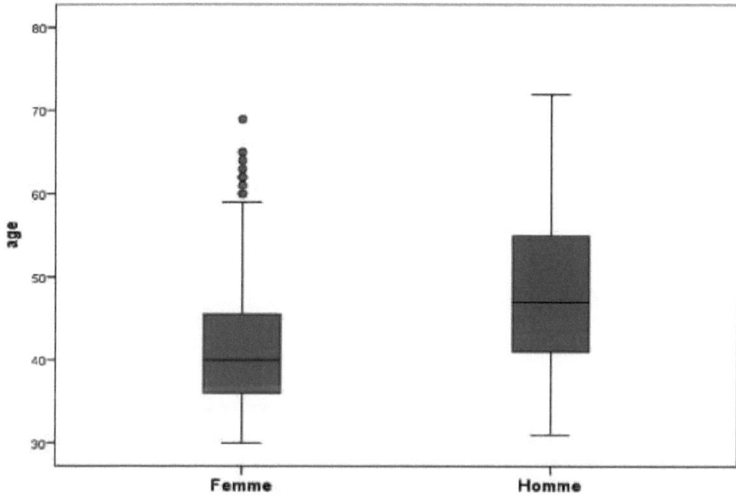

Figure 1. Box plot of participants' age by gender (N=243).

The average years of professional experience were 14.3 ± 10.3 years. The majority (67.5%) worked in the public sector and were medical specialists (79%) with a predominance of medical specialities (63.5%). More than half (53.9%) were university hospital doctors. The majority (69.6%) worked between 31 and 50 hours a week.

The socio-professional characteristics of the participants are summarised in Table I.

Table I. Breakdown of study participants by socio-professional socio-professional characteristics (N=243)

Socio-professional status	Number	Percentage (%)
Gender		
Men	104	42,8
Woman	139	57,2
Age categories (years)		
30-39	81	33,3
40-49	89	36,6

> 50	73	30,0
Years of experience		
<5	47	19,3
5-10	69	28,4
>10	127	52,3
Work sector		
Public	164	67,5
Private	79	32,5
Working area		
Urban	233	95,9
Rural	10	4,1
Specialisation		
General practitioner	51	21,0
Specialist	192	79,0
Type of speciality (N=192)		
Medical	122	63,5
Surgical	60	31,3
Biology / fundamental	10	5,2
Hours worked (per week)		

<30177 ,0

31-409539 ,1

41-507430 ,5

51-602911 ,9

>602811 ,5

Most participants (95.9%) had an average or advanced level of computer skills (Figure 2).

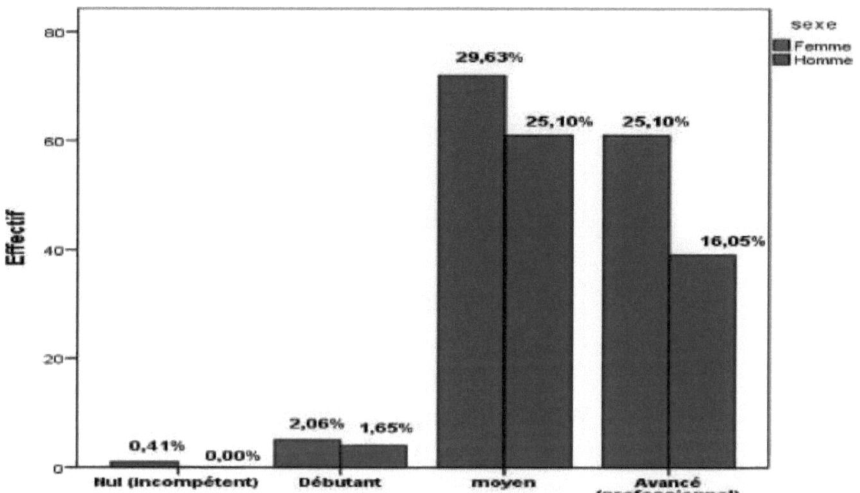

Figure 2. Distribution of computer skills by gender (N=243).

More than half the respondents (53.5%) said they had a good Internet connection at work and a suitable place to practise telemedicine (58%). As for the IT tools available in the workplace, most had access to a computer (86.8%), but more than two-thirds did not have a headset (72.4%) and more than half did not have access to a camera (56.8%) (Figure 3).

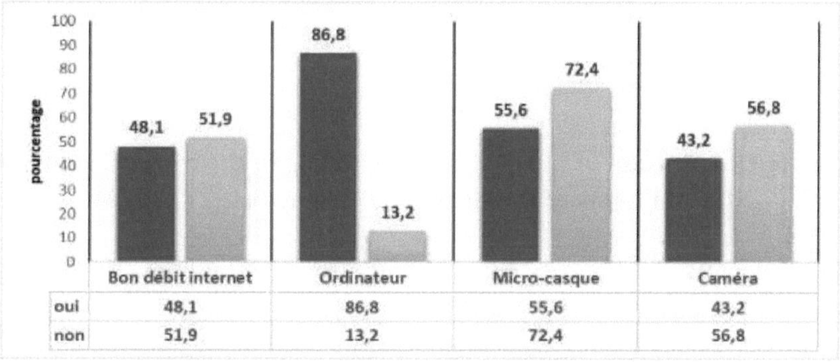

	Bon débit internet	Ordinateur	Micro-casque	Caméra
oui	48,1	86,8	55,6	43,2
non	51,9	13,2	72,4	56,8

Figure 3. Availability of IT tools in the workplace (N=243).

II. Assessment of knowledge

Most of the participants (98.4%, N= 239) had heard of telemedicine, but more than half (56.8%, N= 138) did not know the different areas of its application. Of the 219 respondents to the question on the main sources of information and awareness of telemedicine, the media (television, radio, social media) (32.9%, N=72) or colleagues (26.0%, N=57) were the most frequently cited

(Figure 4).

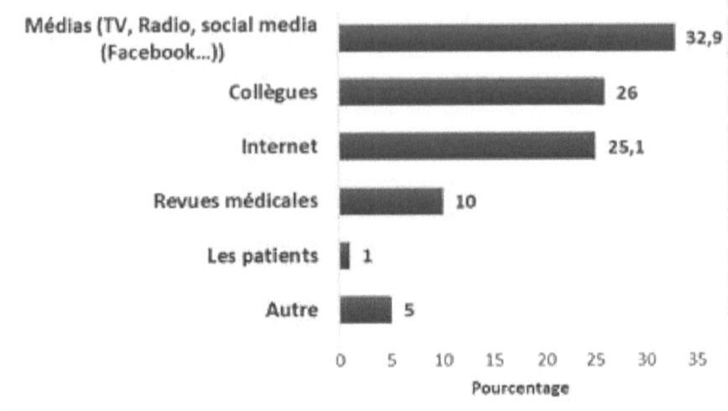

Figure 4. Ways of learning about telemedicine (N=219).

The most common telemedicine activity (63.8%, N=155) was teleconsultation (Figure 5).

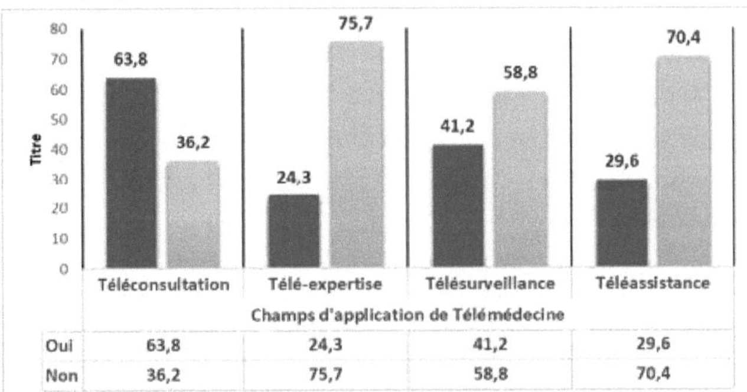

	Téléconsultation	Télé-expertise	Télésurveillance	Téléassistance
Oui	63,8	24,3	41,2	29,6
Non	36,2	75,7	58,8	70,4

Figure 5. Distribution of participants according to their knowledge of the different fields of application of telemedicine (N=243).

Only 95 doctors (39.1%) had heard of the decree setting out the terms and conditions for telemedicine in Tunisia.

Of the 155 doctors who responded to the question "Do you know the telemedicine regulations in Tunisia?", 93 (60%) replied that they knew nothing about the content of the decree (figure 6).

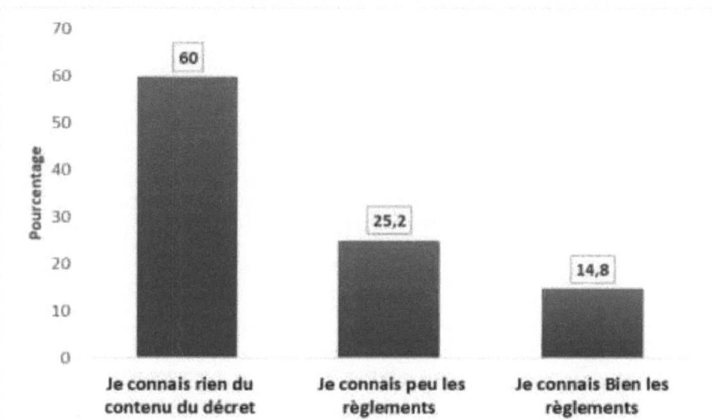

Figure 6. Distribution of participants according to their level of knowledge of the content of the decree setting out the terms and conditions for telemedicine practice in Tunisia (N=155).

The mean value of the knowledge score was 5.2 ± 3.5 points, with extremes ranging from 0 to 12 points (Figure 7).

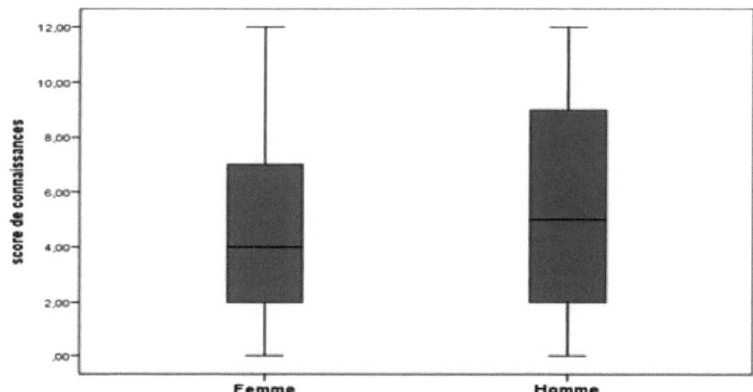

Figure 7. Box plot of participants' knowledge score by gender (N=243).

More than half of the doctors (59.3%; N= 144) had a low level of telemedicine knowledge.

A good level of knowledge was significantly associated with age over 50 (p = 0.02) and years of experience over 10 (p = 0.03) (table II).

Table II. Study of the association between level of knowledge and socio-demographic characteristics of the population studied.

	Level of knowledge		
Features	**Low**	**Good**	**P**

	N (%)	N (%)	
Gender			0,13
Men	56 (53,8)	48 (46,2)	
Woman	88 (63,3)	51 (36,7)	
Age categories (years)			**0,02**
[30-39]	55 (67,9)	26 (32,1)	
[40-49]	55 (61,8)	34 (38,2)	
> 50	34 (46,6)	39 (53,4)	
Years of experience			**0,03**
<5	43 (72,3)	13 (27,7)	
[5-10]	44 (63,8)	25 (36,2)	
>10	66 (52,0)	61 (48,0)	
Work sector			0,4
Public	100 (61,0)	64 (39,0)	
Private	44 (55,7)	35 (44,3)	
Working area			1
Urban	138 (59,2)	95 (40,8)	
Rural	6 (60,0)	4 (40,0)	
Specialisation			0,3
General practitioner	27 (52,9)	24 (47,1)	
Specialist	117 (60,9)	75 (39,1)	
Working hours (per week)			0,07
<30	9 (52,9)	8 (47,1)	
[31-40]	64 (67,4)	31 (32,6)	
[41-50]	41 (55,4)	33 (44,6)	
[51-60]	19 (65,5)	10 (34,5)	
>60	11 (39,3)	17 (60,7)	

III. Assessment of Attitudes

1. Benefits of telemedicine

The mean score for the perceived benefits of telemedicine was 20.1±6 points (total score ranging from 0 to 28). The mean score was significantly higher in men than in women (21.4 vs. 19.2; p=0.004) (Figure 8).

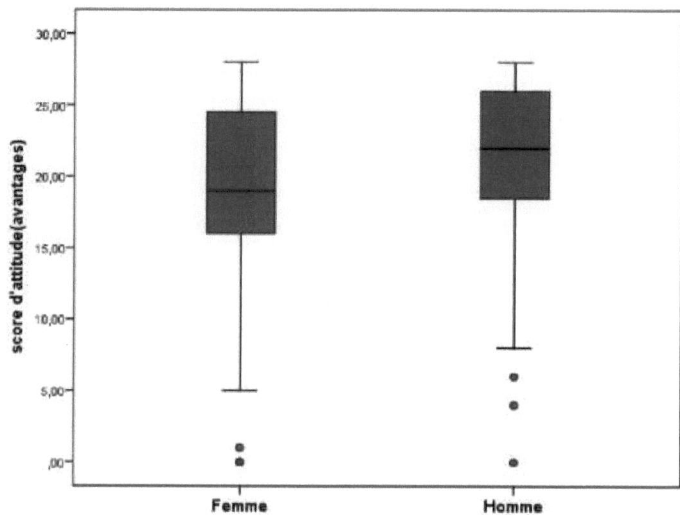

Figure 8. Box plot of telemedicine perceived benefits score by gender (N=243).

The majority of respondents (89.3%) had an average or high score for the benefits they received.

Most participants agreed or strongly agreed that telemedicine was useful for the patient (82.3%, N=200), for the doctor (81.5%, N=198) and for the healthcare system in general (74.5%, N=181).

Most participants agreed or strongly agreed that telemedicine improves access to healthcare (82.3%, N=200) and facilitates communication between healthcare professionals (86.4%, N=210).

In response to the question "What do you think would be the main benefit in your practice of carrying out telemedicine procedures?", doctors cited the benefit for patients (34.2%), telemonitoring (22.2%) and the exchange of opinions and advice between doctors (tele-expertise) (20.6%) (Figure 9).

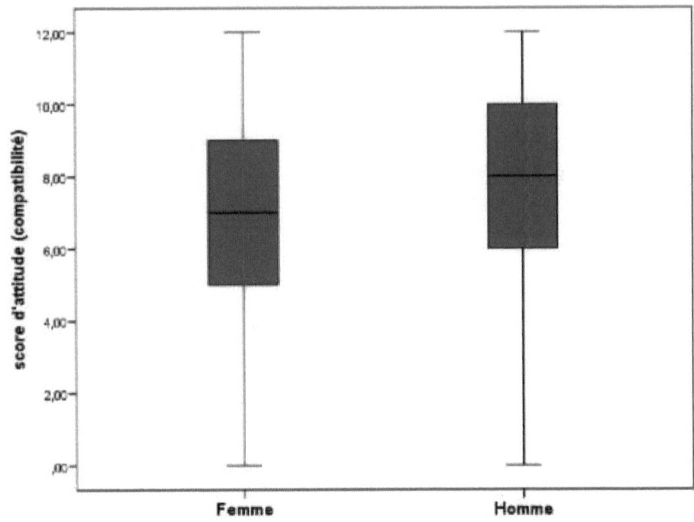

Figure 9. Box plot of lost telemedicine compatibility score by gender (N=243).

Most of the doctors questioned thought that telemedicine represents the future of medical practice (70.8%, N=172), is a necessity (72.0%, N=175), is a hope (70.8%, N=172) and is of interest not only to specialists (84.0%, N=204). The majority (83.5%, N=203) of respondents said they were interested in telemedicine.

2. Compatibility of telemedicine with medical practice doctors

The mean telemedicine lost compatibility score was 7.3 ± 2.8 points (total score ranging from 0 to 12). The mean score was slightly higher in men than in women (7.8 vs. 7.0; p=0.005) (Figure 10).

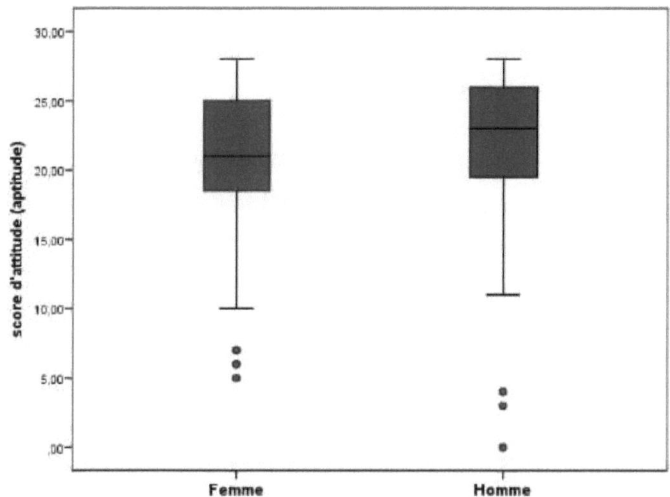

Figure 10. Box plot of aptitude score and willingness to practise telemedicine by gender (N=243).

The majority of respondents (76.5%, N=186) had an average or high score for the degree of lost compatibility of telemedicine with their practice.

2.1. Ability and willingness to try telemedicine

The mean score for aptitude and motivation to try telemedicine (total score ranging from 0 to 28) was 21.5 ± 5.0 points. There was no significant difference in the mean score according to sex (21.9 in men vs. 21.2 in women; p=0.3) (Figure 11).

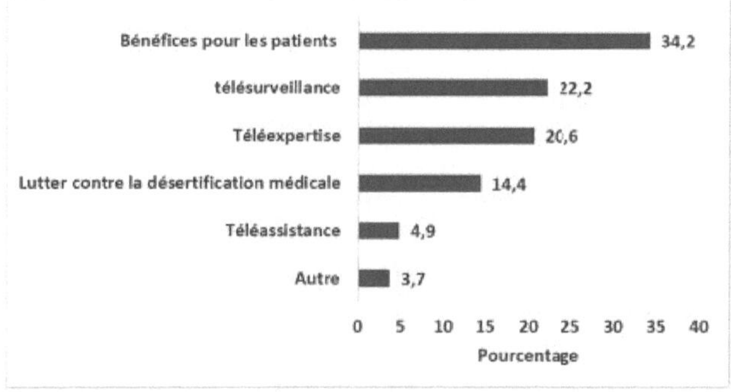

Figure 11. Distribution of participants according to the main benefit received from telemedicine (N=243).

The majority (93%, N=226) had a moderate or high willingness to try telemedicine.

Most participants (86.8%, N=211) agreed or strongly agreed to receive telemedicine training; 78.2% (N=190) thought telemedicine would be useful in their practices and 88.5% (N=215) would agree to use telemedicine in the future.

2.2. Perpetual complexity and disadvantages

The mean score for complexity and perceived inconvenience for telemedicine was 14.8 ± 4.9 points (total score ranging from 0 to 27).

The majority (64.6%, N=157) had a medium or high score for not considering telemedicine complex or inconvenient (Table III).

Table III. Attitudes of doctors towards telemedicine according to perceived benefits, compatibility with their practice, willingness to try, and perceived threats and drawbacks of telemedicine.
practice, willingness to try, and perceived threats and drawbacks of telemedicine (N=243)

Attitude	Strongly disagree N (%)	Disagree N (%)	Don't know (Indecis) N (%)	Agree N (%)	Strongly agree N (%)	Average score Mean ± standard deviation
Benefits						**20,1 ± 6**
Is an intëressante (Useful) practice **for the patient**	6 **(2,5)**	11 **(4,5)**	26 **(10,7)**	88 **(36,2)**	112 **(46,1)**	
Is an interesting (Useful) practice **for the practitioner**	8 **(3,3)**	10 **(4,1)**	27 **(11,1)**	88 **(36,2)**	110 **(45,3)**	
Is an interesting (useful) practice for **the Tunisian health system**	11 **(4,5)**	14 **(5,8)**	37 **(15,2)**	72 **(29,6)**	109 **(44,9)**	
Improving access to healthcare	7 **(2,9)**	11 **(4,5)**	25 **(10,3)**	91 **(37,4)**	109 **(44,9)**	
Reduces the risk of medical error	41 **(16,9)**	57 **(23,5)**	71 **(29,2)**	45 **(18,5)**	29 **(11,9)**	
Facilitates diagnosis and treatment	15 **(6,2)**	44 **(18,1)**	63 **(25,9)**	66 **(27,2)**	55 **(22,6)**	
Facilitates communication between healthcare professionals	5 **(2,1)**	8 **(3,3)**	20 **(8,2)**	89 **(36,6)**	121 **(49,8)**	
Compatibility						**7,3 ± 2,8**
Is compatible with all aspects of my clinical practice	39 **(16,0)**	57 **(23,5)**	70 **(28,8)**	39 **(16,0)**	38 **(15,6)**	
Is compatible with my current professional situation	21 **(8,6)**	32 **(13,2)**	64 **(26,3)**	67 **(27,6)**	59 **(24,3)**	

It would be more useful for monitoring the elderly and chronic illnesses.	7 **(2,9)**	12 **(4,9)**	42 **(17,3)**	100 **(41,2)**	82 **(33,7)**	
Ability/willingness to try telemedicine						**21,5 ± 5**
I would like to be trained in this practice	4 **(1,6)**	6 **(2,5)**	22 **(9,1)**	79 **(32,5)**	132 **(54,3)**	
It's necessary (or useful) to use tëlëmëdecine in my daily practice	7 **(2,9)**	15 **(6,2)**	31 **(12,8)**	82 **(33,7)**	108 **(44,4)**	
The trial of an application of tëlëmëdecine is an opportunity to be seized	4 **(1,6)**	8 **(3,3)**	26 **(10,7)**	93 **(38,3)**	112 **(46,1)**	
A simple trial of a telemedicine application is all that's needed to assess this.	18 **(7,4)**	64 **(26,3)**	95 **(39,1)**	42 **(17,3)**	24 **(9,9)**	
I'm willing to try out a telemedicine application (an exercise) before using it.	5 **(2,1)**	5 **(2,1)**	14 **(5,8)**	105 **(43,2)**	114 **(46,9)**	
I am open to (I accept) the use of telemedicine	4 **(1,6)**	3 **(1,2)**	21 **(8,6)**	102 **(42,0)**	113 **(46,5)**	
It is necessary and useful to create a structure dedicated to the practice of telemedicine in each hospital.	4 **(1,6)**	9 **(3,7)**	30 **(12,3)**	76 **(31,3)**	124 **(51,0)**	
Threats / Complexity / Drawbacks						**14,8 ± 4,9**
Requires too much mental effort	24 **(9,9)**	60 **(24,7)**	77 **(31,7)**	70 **(28,8)**	12 **(4,9)**	
Would be difficult for me **to learn**	4 **(1,6)**	17 **(7,0)**	50 **(20,6)**	106 **(43,6)**	66 **(27,2)**	
Would be difficult to **apply and use** for me	10 **(4,1)**	19 **(7,8)**	62 **(25,5)**	98 **(40,3)**	54 **(22,2)**	
Increases workload	19 **(7,8)**	56 **(23,0)**	91 **(37,4)**	52 **(21,4)**	25 **(10,3)**	
Constitutes a **threat** to the practice of medicine for the practitioner	14 **(5,8)**	36 **(14,8)**	87 **(35,8)**	75 **(30,9)**	31 **(12,8)**	
Involves the **medico-legal responsibility** of the doctor who is not covered by a law protecting his rights	89 **(36,6)**	77 **(31,7)**	61 **(25,1)**	11 **(4,5)**	5 **(2,1)**	
Is a threat to patient	29	54	81	54	25	

confidentiality and privacy	**(11,9)**	**(22,2)**	**(33,3)**	**(22,2)**	**(10,3)**

Perceived obstacles to the application of telemedicine in doctors' practices

The main obstacles and disincentives to telemedicine implementation were: organisational and implementation difficulties (84%, N=204), incomplete examination of patients (80. 7%, N=196), high costs (80.7% , N=196), lack of training (80.7% , N=196), and lack of resources (80.7% , N=196).
(79.8%, N=194) and the medicolegal aspect (79.8%, N=194) (Figure 12).

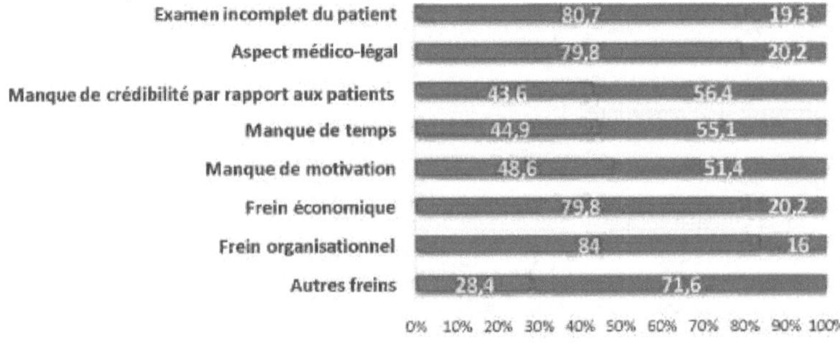

Figure 12. Main obstacles to the application of telemedicine

(N=243).

The study of the association between the various obstacles cited to the application of telemedicine in Tunisia and the socio-professional factors of the study population is shown in Table IV.

Table IV. Identification of the main obstacles, perceived by doctors, to the application of telemedicine and study of their association with the socio-professional factors of the study population

application of telemedicine and study of their association with the socio-professional factors of the study population (N=243)

	Obstacles to the application of telemedecine			
Socio-economic factors professionals	**Organisational brake**			
	YES N (%)	**NO** N (%)	**OR** [IC95%]	**p**
Gender				0,4
Men	85 (81,7)	19 (18,3)	0,75 [0,4 -1,5]	

Woman	119 (85,6)	20 (14,4)		
Age categories				0,18
30-39	72 (88,9)	9 (11,1)	-	
40-49	70 (78,7)	19 (21,3)		
> 50	62 (84,9)	11 (15,1)		
Years of experience				0,12
<5	44 (93,6)	3 (6,4)	-	
5-10	57 (82,6)	12 (17,4)		
>10	103 (81,1)	24 (18,9)		
Work sector				**$<10^{-3}$**
Public	151 (92,1)	13 (7,9)	5,7 [2,7 -11,9]	
Privu	53 (67,1)	26 (32,9)		
Working area				1
Urban	195 (83,7)	38 (16,3)	0,6 [0,07 -4,6]	
Rural	9 (90,0)	1 (10,0)		
Specialisation				0,7
Mëdecine дёпёгак	42 (82,4)	9 (17,6)	1,2 [0,5 - 2,6]	
Spë specialist	162 (84,4)	30 (15,6)		
	Economic brake			
	YES	**NO**	**OR**	**p**
Gender				0,2
Men	79 (76,0)	25 (24,0)	0,6 [0,4 - 1,2]	
Woman	115 (82,7)	24 (17,3)		
Age categories				0,6
30-39	67 (82,7)	14 (17,3)	-	
40-49	69 (77,5)	20 (22,5)		
> 50	58	15		

	(79,5)	(20,5)		
Years of experience				0,2
<5	39 (83,0)	8 (17,0)	-	
5-10	59 (85,5)	10 (14,5)		
>10	96 (75,6)	31 (24,4)		
Work sector				**0,001**
Public	141 (86,0)	23 (14,0)	3,0 [1,6 -5,7]	
Privr	53 (67,1)	26 (32,9)		
Working area				0,2
Urban	184 (79,0)	49 (21,0)	-	
Rural	10 (100,0)	0 (0,0)		
Specialisation				0,7
Mëdecine дёпёгак	40 (78,4)	11 (21,6)	1,1 [0,5 - 2,4]	
Spë specialist	154 (80,2)	38 (19,8)		
	Lack of motivation			
	YES	**NO**	**OR**	**P**
Gender				0,7
Men	49 (47,1)	55 (52,9)	0,9 [0,6 -1,5]	
Woman	69 (49,6)	70 (50,4)		
Age categories				0,9
30-39	39 (48,1)	42 (51,9)	-	
40-49	42 (47,2)	47 (52,8)		
> 50	37 (50,7)	36 (49,3)		
Years of experience				0,1
<5	18 (38,3)	29 (61,7)	-	
5-10	39 (56,5)	30 (43,5)		
>10	61 (48,0)	66 (52,0)		
Work sector				0,6
Public	78	86	0,9 [0,5 - 1,5]	

	(47,6)	(52,4)		
Privu	40 (50,6)	39 (49,4)		
Working area				0,7
Urban	114 (48,9)	119 (51,1)	1,4 [0,4 -5,2]	
Rural	4 (40,0)	6 (60,0)		
Specialisation				**0,04**
Mëdecine дёпёга1е	31 (60,8)	20 (39,2)	0,5 [0,3 - 1,0]	
Spë specialist	87 (45,3)	105 (54,7)		
	Lack of time			
	YES	**NO**	**OR**	**P**
Gender				**0,02**
Men	38 (36,5)	66 (63,5)	0,6 [0,3 -0,9]	
Woman	71 (51,1)	68 (48,9)		
Age categories				0,7
30-39	35 (43,2)	46 (56,8)	-	
40-49	43 (48,3)	46 (51,7)		
> 50	31 (42,5)	42 (57,5)		
Years of experience				0,8
<5	19 (40,4)	28 (59,6)	-	
5-10	32 (46,4)	37 (53,6)		
>10	58 (45,7)	69 (54,3)		
Work sector				0,07
Public	67 (40,9)	97 (59,1)	0,6 [0,4 - 1,0]	
Private	42 (53,2)	37 (46,8)		
Working area				0,5
Urban	106 (45,5)	127 (54,5)	1,9 [0,5 - 7,7]	
Rural	3 (30,0)	7 (70,0)		
Specialisation				0,5

General medicine	21 (41,2)	30 (58,8)	1,2 [0,6 - 2,3]	
Specialist	88 (45,8)	104 (54,2)		
	Lack of credi	**bility in relation to patients**		
	YES	**NO**	**OR**	**p**
Gender				**0,007**
Men	35 (33,7)	69 (66,3)	0,5 [0,3 - 0,8]	
Woman	71 (51,1)	68 (48,9)		
Age categories				**0,01**
30-39	45 (55,6)	36 (44,4)	-	
40-49	37 (41,6)	52 (58,4)		
> 50	24 (32,9)	49 (67,1)		
Years of experience				0,1
<5	24 (51,1)	23 (48,9)	-	
5-10	34 (49,3)	35 (50,7)		
>10	48 (37,8)	79 (62,2)		
Work sector				0,6
Public	73 (44,5)	91 (55,5)	1,1 [0,6 - 1,9]	
Private	33 (41,8)	46 (58,2)		
Working area				0,1
Urban	99 (42,5)	134 (57,5)	0,3 [0,08 - 1,2]	
Rural	7 (70,0)	3 (30,0)		
Specialisation				0,2
General medicine	26	25	0,7 [0,4 - 1,3]	
	(51,0)	(49,0)		
Spë specialist	80 (41,7)	112 (58,3)		
	Medico-legal aspects			
	YES	**NO**	**OR**	**p**
Gender				0,1
Men	78 (75,0)	26 (25,0)	0,6 [0,3 - 1,1]	

Woman	116 (83,5)	23 (16,5)		
Age categories				0,8
30-39	66 (81,5)	15 (18,5)	-	
40-49	71 (79,8)	18 (20,2)		
> 50	57 (78,1)	16 (21,9)		
Years of experience				0,5
<5	40 (85,1)	7 (14,9)	-	
5-10	53 (76,8)	16 (23,2)		
>10	101 (79,5)	26 (20,5)		
Work sector				0,09
Public	126 (76,8)	38 (23,2)	0,5 [0,3 -1,2]	
Privu	68 (86,1)	11 (13,9)		
Working area				0,7
Urban	186 (79,8)	47 (20,2)	0,9 [0,2 - 4,8]	
Rural	8 (80,0)	2 (20,0)		
Specialisation				0,8
Mëdecine дёпёгак	40 (78,4)	11 (21,6)	1,1 [0,5 - 2,4]	
Spë specialist	154 (80,2)	38 (19,8)		
	Incomplete examination of the patient			
	YES	**NO**	**OR**	**p**
Gender				0,2
Men	80 (76,9)	24 (23,1)	0,7 [0,3 - 1,2]	
Woman	116 (83,5)	23 (16,5)		
Age categories				0,2
30-39	69 (85,2)	12 (14,8)	-	

The doctor's sector of work was significantly associated with citing the organisational barrier as one of the perceived obstacles to the implementation of telemedicine in Tunisia (92.1% of doctors working in the public sector vs. 67.1% of doctors working in the private sector; p<10-3). Similarly, sector of work was significantly associated with economic hindrance (86.0% of doctors working in the public sector vs. 67.1% of doctors working in the private sector; p=0.001). Specialty was significantly associated with the perception of lack of motivation as one of the obstacles to telemedicine practice in Tunisia (60.8% of general practitioners vs. 45.3% of specialists; p=0.04). Lack of time was significantly (p=0.02) more of an obstacle for women (51.1%) than for men (36.5%). Lack of credibility in relation to patients was significantly associated with gender (51.1% of women vs. 33.7% of men; p=0.007) and age category (55.6% in the 30-39 age group; 41.6% in the 40-49 age group; 32.9% in the >50 age group; p=0.01).

IV. Evaluation of practices

Around half (46.9%, n=114) of the doctors surveyed have used telemedicine at least once before (Figure 13), using either the mobile phone (91%) or social media (64%).

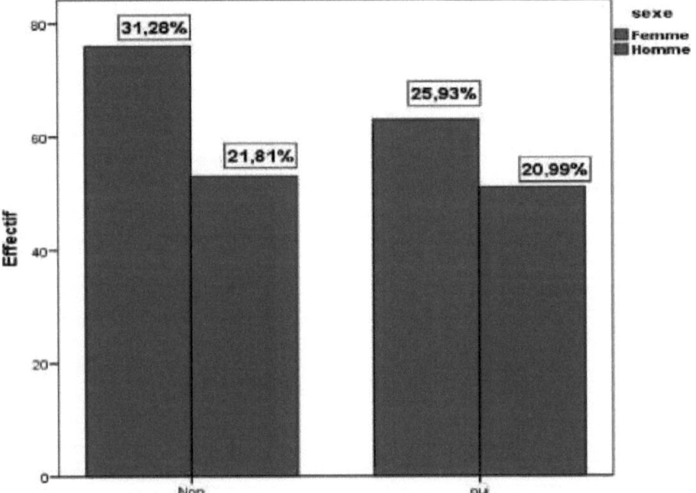

Figure 13. Breakdown of telemedicine use by gender (N=243).

Almost half (44.5%) said they practised telemedicine on a regular basis (Figure 14).

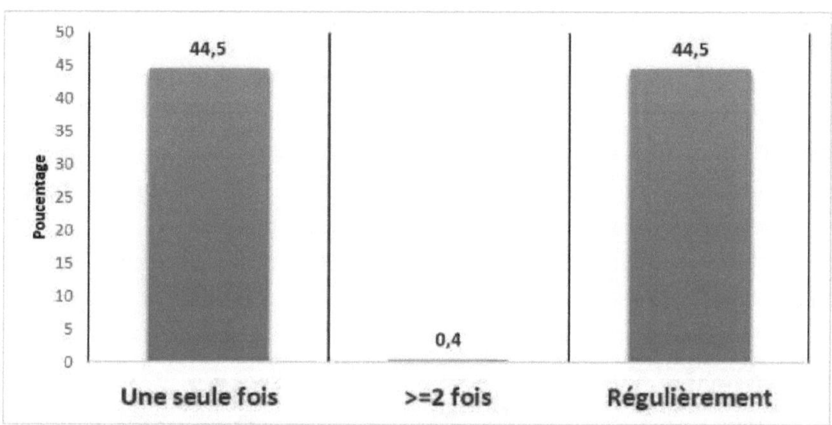

Figure 14. Distribution of doctors who have used telemedicine, by frequency of use (N=110).

The majority of doctors who reported having practised telemedicine, 82.4%, had five or more years of professional experience; 55.3% were women; 59.6% worked in the public sector and 78.9% were specialists. There was no statistically significant association between the socio-professional characteristics of the study population and telemedicine practice.

More than half of those questioned (63.4%) said they intended to use telemedicine in their future activities, and 32.1% were undecided.

4 DISCUSSION

Our study was a descriptive, cross-sectional CAP study involving a sample of 243 Tunisian doctors, who were interviewed online using a Google Forms form. The main aim of our study was to assess the knowledge, attitudes and practices of Tunisian doctors towards telemedicine. The secondary objective was to determine the obstacles to its use in medical practice.

The level of telemedicine knowledge was considered low for more than half of the doctors, with a mean knowledge score of 5.2 ± 3.5 points. A good level of knowledge was significantly associated with an age category of over 50 years and years of experience of over 10 years.

Regarding doctors' attitudes towards telemedicine, the majority scored medium to high on the perceived benefits of telemedicine, such as its usefulness for the patient, the doctor and for the healthcare system in general, the benefit of improving access to healthcare, and the facilitation of communication between healthcare professionals. The majority of doctors had a medium to high score for the degree of lost compatibility of telemedicine with their practice. Most doctors scored moderate to high in their willingness to try telemedicine. Almost two thirds of doctors had a moderate or high score for not seeing telemedicine as complex or inconvenient.

Most of the doctors interviewed believed that telemedicine represents the future of medical practice, that it is a necessity, and that it represents hope for the future of medicine. More than three quarters of those questioned said they were generally interested in telemedicine.

The main barriers and obstacles perceived to the application of telemedicine in doctors' practices were: organisational and implementation difficulties, incomplete examination of patients, economic costs and remuneration, and the medico-legal aspect of telemedicine practice.

Around half of the doctors surveyed have used telemedicine at least once before, using either mobile phones or social media.

As far as we know, our study is the first in Tunisia to assess the level of knowledge, attitudes and practice of doctors towards telemedicine.

The size of our sample was considerable (N=243) and we included all categories of doctors (public or private sector doctors; specialists and non-specialists). All age groups and generations of practising physicians were represented.

Our study was of the CAP type. This type of epidemiological study offers several advantages in the field of public health research. They enable us to understand people's behaviour and practices in relation to certain health problems (such as diseases, risk factors or health interventions). They provide useful and valuable data by measuring the knowledge and attitudes that influence behaviour and practices prior to the planning and implementation of a targeted public health programme or intervention.

By assessing doctors' knowledge of telemedicine, our CAP study has identified gaps in doctors' knowledge of telemedicine. This enables us to target education and communication needs to improve doctors' level of knowledge and raise their awareness of the importance of telemedicine.

By measuring doctors' perceptions and attitudes towards telemedicine, it is possible to design appropriate interventions to promote positive change and ensure the success of the implementation of this new communication technique. It is therefore essential to have a clear idea of the opinion, vision, way of perceiving and degree of acceptability of telemedicine by the main players, namely doctors.

This type of study generates a large database that could serve as a reference for future assessments of the subject. The results of our study can be used to guide new studies or deepen our understanding of telemedicine issues.

In addition, our study enabled us to draw up, in a simple and inexpensive way, an inventory of the level of knowledge of doctors and to measure the degree of acceptance and conviction of doctors and the extent to which they are prepared to accept and practise telemedicine and adopt it in their professional practices. It is also an opportunity to raise awareness of the subject among the doctors surveyed and to encourage them to reflect on and express their opinions and criticisms on the subject.

One of the limitations of our study is that it involved a non-representative sample of Tunisian doctors. Acceptance of participation in the study was purely voluntary. This could introduce a selection bias, as doctors with a positive attitude or favourable prior experience towards telemedicine were perhaps more concerned by the question and more likely to participate. However, we tried to target a very large number of doctors throughout Tunisia by having an almost exhaustive list of emails from doctors registered with the Medical Council as well as an additional list of emails from all university hospital teachers belonging to the Faculty of Medicine in Tunis. Other limitations include the fact that this study was only of interest to doctors. Patients and political decision-makers were not surveyed.

The literature review enabled us to select a number of studies which we considered interesting and which presented a methodology almost similar to our own. Table V summarises these studies in the Maghreb countries, Africa, the Middle East and internationally.

Table V. Summary table of the main studies selected from the literature review

Article and author	Year of publication	Methodology and type of survey	Main results
Study in Ethiopia (12) Kirubel Birouk1and Eden Abetu	2018	A cross-sectional facility-based study was carried out among 312 health professionals working in North Gondar.	Only 37.6% of doctors had a good knowledge of telemedicine, 93.3% agreed or completely agreed to try telemedicine.
Study in India (14)Zayabalaradjane Zayapragassarazan 1, Santosh Kumar 2	2016	Cross-sectional survey	41% had a good knowledge of telemedicine As far as attitudes towards telemedicine are concerned, 39% of respondents have a high positive attitude, while 56% do not have the necessary skills to manage telemedicine and its related equipment. Only 60% of doctors expressed an interest in adopting telemedicine for their future practice,
Study in Iran (15) Abbas Sheikhtaheri 1, Masoumeh Sarbaz 2, Khalil Kimiafar 3, Masoumeh Ghayour 2, Soudabeh Rahmani 2	2016	Cross-sectional descriptive study	The main sources of information about telemedicine were the media (30.3%) and colleagues (51.4%).
Study in Libya (16) Elhadi et al	2021	Cross-sectional study	26.6% had professional IT skills, 67.2% had an average level of IT skills and 6.2% had a beginner level of IT skills.
Study carried out in northern Uganda(17) : Geoffrey Tabo Olok1, Walter Onen Yagos2*and Emilio Ovuga3	2015	Cross-sectional study	57.4% said they had access to a computer and 48.5% had access to the Internet at work The level of skills was moderate (average of 3.66)
Telemedicine experiences in HIV care during the COVID-19(18) pandemic: a mixed-methods study (USA) Dini Harsono 1, Yanhong Deng 2, Sangyun Chung 2	2022	Cross-sectional study	Of the seropositive patients (PWH) surveyed who had a telemedicine appointment (n = 205), 42.4% perceived telemedicine visits as useful during the pandemic. PWH and clinical staff identified benefits of telemedicine: (1) ability to engage and re-engage patients in care; (2) perception of being patient-

			centred and flexible; (3) opportunity to involve family and multidisciplinary care team members; and (4) opportunity to improve mastery of telemedicine use through practice and support. Barriers identified included: (1) technical challenges; (2) confidentiality issues; (3) loss of routine clinical experience and interaction; (4) limited objective remote patient monitoring; and (5) reimbursement issues. Efforts to optimise telemedicine for HIV care should consider strategies to improve technological support for PWH, flexible options for accessing care, additional platforms to enable remote patient monitoring, and appropriate billing and reimbursement methods.
Patient satisfaction with telemedicine in the Philippines during the COVID-19 pandemic (19) Alicia Victoria G. Noceda1*, Lianne Margot M. Acierto1, Morvenn Chaimek C. Bertiz1, David Emmanuel H. Dionisio1, Chelsea Beatrice L. Laurito1, Girard Alphonse T.	2023	Mixed methods study	60% of participants consider it affordable. Patients prefer to use telemedicine when their state of health is not urgent and does not require an in-depth physical examination. Patient satisfaction is influenced by factors such as security against COVID-19, confidentiality of exchanges, and the accessibility and availability of different communication platforms.
Sanchez let Arianna Maever Loreche 1, The qualitative experience of access to	2022	Qualitative study	The transition to telesales has been useful but difficult.
and clinical encounters in Australian healthcare during COVID- 19 (22) Jenifer Blancl*, Julie Byleslet Tom Walley2		interpretative	persistent barriers to the telesante process need to be overcome; face-to-face consultations are essential; changes in workload pressures and the potential for duplication; essential change in working practices;

Telemedicine is increasingly being used to improve healthcare, especially in societies where digitalisation is booming. It plays a crucial role in the transition to telehealth, which aims to manage and support health by integrating telecommunication systems and technologies to protect and improve health (20).

The adoption and use of ICTs in health are faced with various challenges. Among these challenges, human aspects such as users' knowledge and attitude towards technology play a crucial role.

I. Assessing the knowledge and benefits of telemedicine

The results of our study showed that most Tunisian doctors have heard of telemedicine, mainly through the media or through their colleagues. These results are consistent with those of a large survey conducted in European countries (22) and Iran (15).

However, the level of telemedicine knowledge was considered low and unsatisfactory for more than half of the doctors, with only 39.1% of them having heard of the Tunisian telemedicine decree. Our results do not differ greatly from studies published in other developing countries. Indeed, only 37.6% of doctors in Ethiopia had a good knowledge of telemedicine (12). Furthermore, a descriptive study in India obtained similar results (41% had a good level of knowledge) (14). In our study, a good level of knowledge was significantly associated with an age category of over 50 years and years of experience of over 10 years. These results differ from a cross-sectional Indian study that found higher knowledge scores in physicians aged less than 50 years (14). Our results may be explained by the fact that older doctors have accumulated more clinical experience over the years, which enables them to better understand the potential benefits of telemedicine. Their experience can give them a broader perspective on health issues and patient management, and they can identify situations in which telemedicine can be effective and safe. Their in-depth knowledge of medicine in general can also make it easier for them to learn and adapt to new technologies.

Older doctors, particularly those who have been practising for more than 10 years, have seen the problems of access to healthcare evolve. They may have witnessed the decline in the number of doctors in certain regions and the phenomenon of medical deserts. Telemedicine can be seen as a solution to overcoming these challenges by offering a convenient alternative for patients who find it difficult to physically visit a doctor. Older and more experienced doctors may therefore be more inclined to train and use telemedicine to meet their patients' needs.

Research conducted at Michigan State University in the USA, and other similar studies, have highlighted the importance of healthcare professionals' attitudes and perceptions of telemedicine (23-27). Physicians' attitudes towards telemedicine have a significant influence on its adoption and effective implementation. Their perception of the technology, its advantages and disadvantages, and its impact on the quality of care and the doctor-patient relationship play a key role in their perception and adoption.

In our study, most participants had a positive attitude towards telemedicine and its perceived benefits, which is consistent with the results of studies conducted at Michigan State University and in other countries (23,25,28,29).

Among the benefits of telemedicine most frequently mentioned in our study were improving access to healthcare (82.3%) and facilitating communication between healthcare professionals (86.4%).

It is also important to stress that the use of telemedicine, particularly in disadvantaged regions of Tunisia where at least 40% of the population live, can offer many advantages. It helps to improve the availability of high-quality local care and to tackle the shortage of medical staff (30). Telemedicine offers an effective solution for meeting healthcare needs in areas where medical resources are limited. It reduces geographical barriers and improves access to care.

Other benefits of telemedicine discussed in the literature also include promoting cooperation between the public and private sectors (31), reducing lost time and long journeys for patients (32), and solving the problems associated with medical deserts (33,31).

Qualitative studies have also highlighted the economic gains associated with the use of telemedicine (31,34).

The advantages and benefits of telemedicine are numerous for patients, healthcare professionals and the entire healthcare sector in general.

For patients, it reduces costs such as travel associated with traditional consultations. It provides improved access to healthcare for people living in geographically isolated areas, for the elderly, for prisoners, and for others.

vulnerable populations, who can benefit from easier access to healthcare thanks to telemedicine. Remote consultations also enable patients to save time by avoiding journeys to doctors' surgeries or hospitals. They can consult a doctor from their home or workplace, which is particularly practical for busy people or those with reduced mobility. It also enables regular monitoring of patients with chronic illnesses, who can benefit from regular, convenient monitoring via telemedicine, improving their quality of life and their medical care. One of the main benefits for doctors is that it enables them to manage their time more effectively. It means that procedures and activities can be carried out remotely, and patients' condition can be tracked and monitored. It offers the possibility of collaboration and tele-expertise, enabling specialist advice to be sought remotely, facilitating collaboration between general practitioners and specialists. In this way, tele-expertise helps to improve the quality of diagnoses and therapeutic decisions.

A study carried out in the Philippines to assess patient satisfaction with telemedicine found that it is generally well received, with around 60% of participants considering it affordable (19). Patients prefer to use telemedicine when their state of health is not urgent and does not require an in-depth physical examination. Patient satisfaction is influenced by factors such as security against transmissible diseases, as in the case of COVID-19, the confidentiality of exchanges, and the accessibility and availability of different communication platforms. However, some patients who participated in this study expressed concerns about the quality of care and services provided by telemedicine providers, as well as the limitations of telemedicine in terms of diagnosis and management (19).

These results underline the importance of raising doctors' awareness of the benefits of telemedicine in order to encourage more widespread and successful adoption of this innovative practice.

On the other hand, the willingness to explore telemedicine in their future practice was widely expressed by the majority (93%) of our participants. These results differ from those of a cross-sectional survey conducted in India, where only 60% of participants expressed an interest in adopting this new technology in their future careers (14). In contrast, Ethiopian doctors showed greater openness to telemedicine, with 93.3% expressing strong support for the idea of trying it out and 81.9% expressing a desire to use a telemedicine application (12).

These differences can be attributed to cultural differences, the quality of pre-existing healthcare infrastructures and the specific needs of each country.

The positive attitude of Tunisian doctors towards telemedicine reflects their willingness to adopt innovative approaches to improve the quality of healthcare and keep up with advances in modern medicine. In Tunisia, telemedicine has become an essential option in the healthcare sector, particularly in response to the Coxsackie-19 pandemic and the challenges posed by medical deserts and regional disparities in access to care.

This positive view of telemedicine by doctors paves the way for serious investment and wider adoption of this technology in the country. This will provide promising opportunities to improve access to healthcare, strengthen inter-professional collaboration and address the specific challenges associated with the availability of healthcare services in certain regions of Tunisia.

II. Assessment of practices

As far as telemedicine is concerned, almost half of the doctors questioned (46. 9%) have already carried out telemedicine activities,
mainly by using their mobile phone (91%) or social media (64%).
The use of information and communication technologies (ICTs) in the healthcare sector requires the availability of IT tools and a location suitable for telemedicine practice.
With regard to computer skills, the vast majority of participants (95.9%) in our study said they had an average or high level. In contrast, a study conducted in Libya revealed that only 26.6% of participants had professional-level computer skills, while 67.2% had average computer skills and 6.2% had beginner computer skills (16).
We found that the majority of participants in our study had conditions deemed favourable for practising telemedicine. More than half of the participants had a good Internet connection, more than half had a suitable place to practise telemedicine and 86.8% had access to a computer. However, it should be pointed out that a significant number of participants did not have the necessary accessories for remote consultations.
A study carried out in France in 2017 among 278 doctors also highlights this problem. Although 84% of doctors said they had a good Internet connection and 99.6% had access to a computer, only 34% had a space dedicated to telemedicine. Furthermore, few doctors had the essential accessories, with only 36% equipped with a camera and 25% with a headset (33).
These results underline the need to take into account not only the availability of basic technological tools, such as access to the Internet and a computer, but also the specific accessories required for the best conditions for telemedicine practice. It is crucial to guarantee an appropriate and well-equipped environment for doctors to be able to carry out high-quality and effective remote consultations. This issue needs to be addressed in order to facilitate the wider and successful adoption of telemedicine in medical practice.

III. The challenges and limits of telemedicine

Furthermore, telemedicine, as a remote medical practice using digital communication and information solutions, presents challenges and limits.
In our study, we tried to identify the main obstacles to the use of telemedicine by doctors.
It is essential to identify these specific barriers in order to develop effective strategies to promote wider and successful adoption of telemedicine among

physicians.
In Tunisia, the development of telemedicine faces a number of obstacles that need to be overcome if telemedicine is not to remain confined to hospital practice, and if its expansion into the medical field is to be encouraged. These obstacles require efforts to reduce apprehensions and make doctors more aware of the importance of telemedicine.
According to the results of our study, organisational and implementation challenges are the main obstacle (84%) to the development of telemedicine, according to the doctors surveyed.
These findings are in line with several other studies, including one carried out in France (34) and a meta-analysis carried out on Middle Eastern countries (35), which highlighted the significant obstacles imposed by organisational structure, such as infrastructure, professional expertise, strategic planning, training, effective monitoring, as well as representation, insurance and reimbursement issues, which affect the implementation of telemedicine in hospitals in the region (35).
The organisational barrier also includes the fear linked to technical problems, such as the importance of developing a high-speed connection, questions of data reliability and security (37), and the absence of secure messaging in medical practices (36). All of these factors raise concerns about confidentiality and give rise to worries among doctors about their ability to adapt to and master these technologies. The risks of technical failure and concerns about the reliability of the new technologies and liability have also been reported (31,34). It is therefore necessary to resolve these various technical issues in order to optimise the development of telemedicine.
According to the results of our study, the incomplete examination of patients is also a major obstacle for the doctors surveyed. Indeed, the fear of not being able to carry out a physical examination has been reported in many other studies (24,32,37). Preserving the patient's place and maintaining the quality of the doctor-patient relationship (37), avoiding loss of information due to lack of direct contact (24,37) and preventing dehumanisation are essential concerns for doctors. The privileged relationship between the attending physician and his patient is considered essential, as it enables better patient management by not overlooking any non-verbal diagnostic elements and by promoting clear communication. However, information and communication technologies (ICTs) are already present in the doctor-patient relationship, with many patients using the Internet for information, which may influence their perceptions of their pathologies and treatment (32,37).

In addition, the economic cost and remuneration barrier was identified as one of the main obstacles to the development of telemedicine in our study. The investment required in new equipment, the lack of clear remuneration for doctors (31) and the reluctance of health insurers to accept telemedicine have also been mentioned in other studies (34). Moreover, patients may also have economic concerns (34). It is therefore crucial to find public funding to support the development and maintenance of telemedicine practice, so as not to impose additional costs on doctors who are already financially strained, while at the same time clarifying and codifying the details of pricing and the methods of payment for telemedicine procedures within a transparent legal framework.

Other major issues relating to the use and practice of telemedicine include medical and legal liability. Medical professionals carrying out telemedicine procedures must be legally entitled to exercise their profession and be covered by professional indemnity insurance. They must also respect patients' rights and inform them of the benefits and risks associated with a medical procedure, even if it is carried out via telemedicine.

All these results underline the importance of taking all these obstacles into account in order to develop appropriate solutions and encourage the adoption and practice of telemedicine under optimum conditions.

IV. Legal and ethical aspects of telemedicine

In addition, the legal aspect of telemedicine is very important to consider. It is of great importance for the implementation of telemedicine in Tunisia. The establishment of a clear and precise regulatory framework is essential to provide a framework for this practice and guarantee its legality and safety. Fortunately, Tunisia has made significant progress in this area.

The Tunisian Council of Ministers, meeting on 3 March 2022, adopted a decree governing the general conditions for the practice of telemedicine and the areas of its application. This Presidential Decree n°318/2022, published in the Journal Officiel de la Republique Tunisienne on 12 April 2022, establishes a clear legal framework for the practice of telemedicine in Tunisia (13). It sets out the conditions under which telemedicine may be practised, the authorisation procedures, the terms and conditions of agreements between telemedicine platforms and healthcare professionals, and the rules governing data protection and IT security.

Thanks to this decree, telemedicine is now legal in Tunisia, offering numerous advantages. Telemedicine eliminates the need for patients to travel,

facilitates telemonitoring at home or in hospital, and helps to solve the problem of medical deserts by ensuring equitable access to care throughout the country. However, it should be noted that prior authorisation is required, and the Ministry of Health plays a key role in assessing and approving applications for telemedicine authorisation (13).
The Presidential Decree also stipulates that data processed as part of telemedicine procedures must be hosted and stored in Tunisia by a local cloud and hosting service provider, in compliance with current IT security legislation. This is to ensure the confidentiality and protection of patient data.
This decree defines the areas of application of telemedicine as follows (13):

- Teleconsultation: 1 of the acts whereby a doctor or dentist gives a remote medical consultation to a patient, possibly assisted by a qualified health professional.
- Tele-expertise: 1 act whose purpose is to enable a doctor or dentist to seek the opinion of one or more colleagues from a distance, by virtue of their training or particular skills, on the basis of medical information relating to the care of a patient.
- Medical telemonitoring: the act of enabling a doctor or dentist to remotely monitor and interpret the data required for a patient's medical follow-up and, where appropriate, to make decisions relating to the patient's care. The recording and transmission of data may be automated or carried out by the patient themselves or by a healthcare professional.
- Medical teleassistance: the act of enabling a doctor or dentist to provide remote assistance to another healthcare professional when carrying out a medical procedure.
- Medical regulation: the remote medical response provided to a patient as part of the medical triage carried out by the emergency medical assistance services in order to determine and initiate the response best suited to the nature of the call.

The ethical aspect must also be taken into consideration. It plays a very important role in the practice of telemedicine. In our study, the doctors who practised telemedicine mainly used mobile phones or social networks. However, this use raises issues of ethics and confidentiality of patient data.
The Presidential Decree and the National Authority for the Protection of Personal Data (13,38) specify the importance of respecting medical confidentiality and securing and protecting patients' personal data. Patients have the right to medical confidentiality, which means protecting their personal data and respecting their privacy (39).

This Tunisian law defines the telemedicine platform as "a bouquet of digital services grouped together in a common space in compliance with the rules of urbanisation, interoperability, security and ethics, enabling the use of value-added services in the field of telemedicine".

According to this decree, the telemedicine platform must be set up in compliance with the rules governing the identification of the patient and those involved in the telemedicine procedure, the confidentiality and integrity of information exchanges and the traceability of all information relating to the telemedicine procedure, and the retention of personal data for at least ten years. Access to information relating to telemedicine is provided by duly qualified control and inspection bodies. Changes to the data available on the network can be easily traced by the IT centre attached to the Ministry of Public Health. This guarantees optimum operation of the infrastructure. (13).

V. Tunisia's experience and track record in telemedicine

Tunisia has made progress in the field of telemedicine in recent years. The first experience of telemedicine in Tunisia dates back to 1996, when the Ministry of Public Health introduced telemedicine as a working tool as part of its strategic IT plan (40).

Since then, Tunisia has developed regional telemedicine networks which have succeeded in interconnecting local and regional services, thereby promoting this new way of practising conventional medicine (40).

It should be noted that the practice of telemedicine in Tunisia has been legalised thanks to the adoption of a decree governing the general conditions for its exercise and the areas of its application by the Council of Ministers in March 2022 (41).

This legalisation has paved the way for wider use of telemedicine in the country.

There are currently two main telemedicine platforms in Tunisia:

- The Tobba.tn website (42): which enables users to consult doctors online. It offers four main services, namely remote medical consultations via secure video calls, a medical social network, online medical records and a free health space providing simplified answers to questions from the general public. This platform was launched by the ACT start-up in May 2019. It has been authorised by the French National Data Protection Authority (INPDP) under no. 19/02-4264 to process personal health data.
- The Med.tn site (43), which essentially offers an online service for making appointments with healthcare professionals in Tunisia. It also offers

patients the opportunity to interact with doctors about health problems.
In addition, a Tunisian Telemedicine and e-Health Society was officially created in September 2000 with the aim of promoting telemedicine in Tunisia (40).
The company's main tasks were
- Promoting telemedicine in Tunisia.
- Establishing relations with similar associations around the world.
- Collaboration with scientific associations and medical institutions to promote the adoption and integration of telemedicine

In Tunisia, telemedicine is expected to improve access to care, combat regional health disparities and help resolve the health crisis linked to the lack of healthcare professionals and their unbalanced distribution across the country. This opens up the possibility of providing quality local healthcare services on an equitable basis throughout Tunisia (41).

VI. Recommendations and outlook

In the light of all these results, we propose that the way forward should be to study the various aspects of telemedicine in greater depth, and to obtain the opinions and different points of view of the various stakeholders, i.e. political decision-makers, platform managers, doctors and patients. Our study approached the issue of telemedicine from the point of view of doctors only. Targeting patients and policy makers and getting their perceptions and views on telemedicine could be the subject of further studies in order to have a global vision and understanding on the issue with the opinions of all stakeholders.
It would also be very interesting to carry out qualitative studies using interviews or focus groups in order to tackle the subject of telemedicine in greater depth, and why not get the opinions of experts on the advantages and disadvantages of adopting this new technology in the medical field and the various practical ways of implementing it, before embarking on this experiment in order to guarantee the best possible success and profitability for this health project.
Our CAP study identified gaps in doctors' knowledge of telemedicine. This allows us to target education and communication needs, and to set up continuing professional development programmes to improve doctors' knowledge and awareness of telemedicine. These programmes can include interactive sessions, practical workshops and e-learning modules, enabling doctors to acquire the knowledge and skills they need to use telemedicine

effectively.
Furthermore, IT skills are very important for the implementation of the use of telemedicine services. We therefore recommend training programmes in software and IT skills for doctors new to telemedicine technology, particularly in developing countries.
Secondly, it is crucial to improve the technological infrastructure needed to implement telemedicine in Tunisia. This means investing in the extension of Internet connectivity, particularly in rural and underserved areas, to ensure reliable access to telemedicine services. At the same time, cybersecurity needs to be strengthened to protect patient data and guarantee the confidentiality of their information.
the trust needed to encourage the adoption of telemedicine.
The development of clear guidelines and protocols is another important recommendation. These will serve as a reference to guide doctors in using telemedicine effectively and ethically.
Finally, it is essential to encourage research and innovation in the field of telemedicine in Tunisia. The creation of research centres dedicated to telemedicine can also stimulate the exploration of new opportunities and applications. These research initiatives will contribute to the continuous improvement of telemedicine practice, to the resolution of challenges specific to the Tunisian context and to the implementation of new solutions to improve the effectiveness and quality of remote healthcare.
To implement telemedicine in developing countries in general and in Tunisia more specifically, we need to :

- Be familiar with existing programmes in other countries that have successfully used telemedicine and learn from these experiences.
- Overcoming financial challenges and finding financing solutions such as public-private or international partnerships.
- Raising awareness and training healthcare professionals and users in the appropriate use of telemedicine are essential to ensure its acceptance and effective use.
- The problem of limited healthcare infrastructure can present a major challenge to the implementation of telemedicine. It is crucial to assess existing infrastructures and identify technology and connectivity needs. Investment in communications infrastructure, Internet access and medical information systems may be required to support telemedicine.

Finally, telemedicine regulations and policies must be developed and implemented to protect patient confidentiality and ensure quality of care. It is important to comply with health data confidentiality standards and to establish clear guidelines on the use of telemedicine.

5 CONCLUSIONS

elemedicine developed rapidly, particularly during the health crisis linked to the COVID-19 pandemic, which made it possible to Ж standardise the use of telemedicine, in particular the use of the
teleconsultation.

The digitisation of healthcare and telemedicine offer new possibilities and alternatives to traditional medicine, making healthcare more accessible and responding to the current challenges facing healthcare systems.

The main aim of our work was to assess the knowledge, attitudes and practice of Tunisian doctors towards telemedicine. The secondary objective was to determine the obstacles to its use in medical practice.

To meet these objectives, we conducted a descriptive cross-sectional Knowledge, Attitudes and Practice (KAP) study during October 2022. Data was collected online using a Google Forms form that was emailed to a large sample of physicians. We included in our study qualified Tunisian doctors practising in Tunisia, whether in the public or private sector and whatever their specialities. We did not include in our study doctors in training (such as interns or residents).

An introductory email explaining the framework of the study and its main objective was sent, stating that the data would be treated confidentially and anonymously.

The data was collected using a standardised Google Forms questionnaire based on the participants' own responses.

The questionnaire consisted of three main parts relating to the assessment of knowledge, attitudes and practices.

The section assessing attitudes has been subdivided into three sub-sections assessing the perceived benefits of telemedicine, the degree of its compatibility with doctors' practices and the perceived complexity and inconvenience.

A knowledge score was calculated as well as a score for each part relating to attitudes.

The total number of doctors taking part in the study was 243. More than half were female. The age of the participants ranged from 30 to 72 years, with an average of 45 ± 9.6 years.

The average years of professional experience were 14.3 ± 10.3 years. The majority of participants worked in the public sector and were medical specialists with a predominance of medical specialities.

Most of the participants had heard of telemedicine. The best-known telemedicine activity was teleconsultation. Only 39.1% of doctors had heard of the decree setting out the terms and conditions for telemedicine in Tunisia.
Regarding the assessment of knowledge, more than half of the doctors (59.3%) had a low level of telemedicine knowledge. A good level of knowledge was significantly associated with age over 50 years ($p = 0.02$) and years of experience over 10 years ($p = 0.03$).
Regarding the evaluation of attitudes, the majority of respondents (89.3%) had an average or high score for perceived benefits.
Most participants agreed or strongly agreed that telemedicine is useful for the patient, for the doctor and for the healthcare system in general. More than three quarters of respondents had a moderate or high score for the degree of lost compatibility of telemedicine with their practice. The majority (93%) had a moderate or high willingness to try telemedicine. Almost two thirds (64.6%) had a moderate or high score for not considering telemedicine to be complex or inconvenient.
In terms of re-evaluating practices, around half (46.9%) of the doctors surveyed had used telemedicine at least once before, using either the mobile phone or social media. More than half of those surveyed (63.4%) said they intended to use telemedicine in their future activities.
The main obstacles and barriers to telemedicine implementation were organisational and implementation difficulties, incomplete examination of patients, economic costs and remuneration, and the medicolegal aspect.
In the light of these results, we can conclude that despite an insufficient level of knowledge about telemedicine, the doctors surveyed had an overall positive attitude towards the practice of telemedicine. On the other hand, our results indicate that much remains to be done to raise awareness and educate health professionals in general about telemedicine in order to lay the foundations for successful and sustainable adoption of the technology in the country.
Tunisia will be able to make significant progress in the integration and effective use of telemedicine. The regulation of telemedicine practice in Tunisia is a major achievement and a solid starting point for its implementation. Telemedicine will make it possible to break down spatial and temporal barriers to healthcare provision. Its adoption will make it possible to offer high-quality, local health services to all Tunisian citizens, reduce health disparities and combat medical deserts and the lack of health professionals in certain disadvantaged and under-resourced regions. It will

also make it possible to manage the problems associated with budgetary constraints.
On the other hand, there are limits to the implementation of telemedicine in countries with limited resources such as Tunisia, such as technical problems and a defective healthcare infrastructure limiting its potential for rapid and innovative reform.
It is crucial to have a technological and IT infrastructure and good Internet coverage throughout the country in order to support the development of this technology and ensure that it is used and applied in the best possible conditions.
It is also essential that political decision-makers, the Ministry of Health and the Ministry of Information and Communication Technologies are committed to this project and adopt and support the foundations of telemedicine in Tunisia in order to guarantee its success and sustainability.
In this world full of digitalisation and artificial intelligence, which is evolving at a very fast pace, we need to keep up with everything that is new and advanced in the medical field. But we need to adopt a balanced approach to these new technologies and use them with caution and moderation, while maintaining a critical eye. The patient's interests and confidentiality must come first.
Finally, it is essential to remember that telemedicine must respect the ethical and deontological principles governing medical practice in general.

6 REFERENCES

1. **Waller M, Stotler C.** Telemedicine: a Primer. *Curr Allergy Asthma Rep 2018;18(10):54.*

2. **World Health Organization.** Telemedicine: opportunities and developments in member states: report on the second global survey on ehealth 2009. Global observatory for ehealth series, volume 2. *Geneva: WHO; 2010.*

3. **Baker J, Stanley A.** Telemedicine technology: A review of services, equipment, and other aspects. *Curr Allergy Asthma Rep 2018;18(11):60.*

4. **World Health Organization.** Telemedicine. *[Online]. 2022 [Accessed 15/07/2023], availablea the URL: https://www.who.int/goe/publications/ goe_telemedicine_2010.pdf*

5. **Martin-Khan M, Freeman S, Adam K, Betkus G.** The evolution of telehealth. In: Marston HR, Freeman S, Musselwhite C, editors. Mobile e-Health. *Cham Springer; 2017.p.173-98.*

6. **Marshall S, Nerwich N, van Straten C, Petersen L.** Improving healthcare in remote environments via a new integrated, online communication platform. *J Int Soc Telemed eHealth 2017;5:33-1.*

7. **Vatn0y TK, Thygesen E, Dale B.** Telemedicine to support coping resources in home-living patients diagnosed with chronic obstructive pulmonary disease: Patients' experiences. *J Telemed Telecare 2017;23:126-32.*

8. **Haute Autorite de Sante.** Efficience de la telemedecine: état des lieux de la litterature internationale et cadre d'évaluation. Recommandation en sante publique. *Paris: HAS; 2013.*

9. **Reach G.** Has telemedicine become the future of personal medicine? Reflections of a resident at the time of COVID. *Med Mal Metab 2020;14:286-9.*

10. **Petit A, Martin L, Penso-Assathiany D, Consoli S, Assouly P, Velter C, et al.** L'apres Covid-19: vers une dermatologie nouvelle? *Ann Dermatol Venereol 2020;147:411-412.*

11. **Wamala DS, Augustine K.** A meta-analysis of telemedicine success in Africa. *J Pathol Inform 2013;4:6.*

12. **Biruk K, Abetu E.** Knowledge and attitude of health professionals toward telemedicine in resource-limited settings: a cross-sectional study in North West Ethiopia. *J Healthc Eng 2018;2018:2389268.*

13. **Republic of Tunisia.** Decret Presidentiel n° 2022-318 du 8 avril 2022, fixant les conditions generales d'exercice de la telemedecine et les domaines de son application. *JORT No. 40 of 12 April 2022.*

14. **Zayapragassarazan Z, Kumar S.** Awareness, knowledge, attitude and skills of telemedicine among health professional faculty working in teaching

hospitals. *J Clin Diagn Res 2016;10(3):JC01-4.*
15. **Sheikhtaheri A, Sarbaz M, Kimiafar K, Ghayour M, Rahmani S.** Awareness, attitude and readiness of clinical staff towards telemedicine: a study in Mashhad, Iran. *Stud Health Technol Inform 2016;228:142-6.*
16. **Elhadi M, Elhadi A, Bouhuwaish A, Bin Alshiteewi F, Elmabrouk A, Alsuyihili A, et al.** Telemedicine awareness, knowledge, attitude, and skills of health care workers in a low-resource country during the COVID-19 pandemic: cross-sectional study. *J Med Internet Res 2021;23:e20812.*
17. **Olok GT, Yagos WO, Ovuga E.** Knowledge and attitudes of doctors towards ehealth use in healthcare delivery in government and private hospitals in Northern Uganda: a cross-sectional study. *BMC Med Inform Decis Mak 2015;15:87.*
18. **Harsono D, Deng Y, Chung S, Barakat LA, Friedland G, Meyer JP, et al.** Experiences with Telemedicine for HIV Care During the COVID-19 Pandemic: A Mixed-Methods Study. *AIDS Behav 2022;26:2099-111.*
19. **Noceda AV, Acierto LM, Bertiz MC, Dionisio DE, Laurito CB, Sanchez GA, et al.** Patient satisfaction with telemedicine in the Philippines during the COVID- 19 pandemic: a mixed methods study. *BMC Health Serv Res 2023;23:277.*
20. **White J, Byles J, Walley T.** The qualitative experience of telehealth access and clinical encounters in Australian healthcare during COVID-19: implications for policy. *Health Res Policy Syst 2022;20:9.*
21. **World Health Organization.** A health telematics policy in support of WHO's Health-for-all strategy for global health development: report of the WHO Group Consultation on Health Telematics, 11-16 December, Geneva, 1997. *Geneva: WHO; 1998.*
22. **Mairinger T, Gabl C, Derwan P, Ferrer-Roca O, Mikuz G.** What do physicians think of telemedicine? A survey in different European regions. *J Telemed Telecare 1996;2:50-6.*
23. **Whitten P, Holtz B, Nguyen L.** Keys to a successful and sustainable telemedicine program. *Int J Technol Assess Health Care 2010;26:211-6.*
24. **Presseau J, Sniehotta FF, Francis JJ, Campbell NC.** Multiple goals and time constraints: perceived impact on physicians' performance of evidence-based behaviours. *Implement Sci 2009;4:77.*
25. **Angood PB.** Telemedicine, the Internet, and world wide web: overview, current status, and relevance to surgeons. *World J Surg 2001;25:1449-57.*
26. **Lonergan PE, Iii SW, Branagan L, Gleason N, Pruthi RS, Carroll PR, et al.** Rapid utilization of telehealth in a comprehensive cancer center as a response to COVID-19: cross-sectional analysis. *J Med Internet Res 2020;22:e19322.*

27. **Xu H, Huang S, Qiu C, Liu S, Deng J, Jiao B, et al. Monitoring and management** of home-quarantined patients with COVID-19 using a wechat-based telemedicine system: retrospective cohort study. *J Med Internet Res 2020;22:e19514.*
28. **Ayatollahi H, Sarabi FP, Langarizadeh M.** Clinicians' knowledge and perception of telemedicine technology. *Perspect Health Inf Manag 2015;12:1c.*
29. **Barton PL, Brega AG, Devore PA, Mueller K, Paulich MJ, Floersch NR, et al.** Specialist physicians' knowledge and beliefs about telemedicine: a comparison of users and nonusers of the technology. *Telemed J E Health 2007;13:487-99.*
30. **Driss A.** Soutien de 1 Union europeenne au secteur de la sante en Tunisie. Telemedicine as a good practice to alleviate the shortage of specialist doctors in disadvantaged regions in Tunisia. *[Online]. 2022 [Accessed 15/05/2023], availablea the URL: http://www.santetunisie.rns.tn/images/ docs/anis/actualite/2018/avril/paz2/Article-4---La-tlmdecine-_valuation-PAZD-II.pdf*
31. **Lombardo F.** La telemedecine en medecine generale : évaluation du point de vue et du ressenti des medecins generalistes [These]. *Paris: Universite Paris 6, Faculte de Medecine; 2013.*
32. **Mathieu S.** La teleconsultation: 1'avis des medecins generalistes dans les Alpes Maritimes [These]. *Nice: Universite de Nice-Sophia Antipolis, Faculte de Medecine; 2012.*
33. **Messon T.** What is the role of general practitioners in the development of telemedicine? Enquete aupres des medecins generalistes de Gironde [These]. *Bordeaux: Universite de Bordeaux, Faculte de Medecine; 2017.*
34. **Carre E.** Telemedecine: representations et experiences des medecins generalistes: Etude qualitative mènee aupres de medecins generalistes du Languedoc-Roussillon [These]. *Montpellier: Universite de Montpellier I, Faculte de Medecine; 2013.*
35. **Al-Samarraie H, Ghazal S, Alzahrani AI, Moody L.** Telemedicine in Middle Eastern countries: Progress, barriers, and policy recommendations. *Int J Med Inform 2020;141:104232.*
36. **Haw-Shing L.** Programme "Telemedecine en EHPAD " en Gironde : enquete de satisfaction en medecine generale [These]. *Bordeaux: Universite de Bordeaux 2, Faculte de Medecine; 2016.*
37. **Durupt M, Bouchy O, Christophe S, Kivits J, Boivin JM.** Telemedicine in rural areas: representations and experiences of general practitioners. *Sante Publique 2016;28:487-97.*
38. **Ministry of Public Health.** Programme de Developpement de la "Sante

Numerique" en Tunisie 2020. *[En Ligne]. 2020 [Accessed 15/07/2023], available at URL: http://www.santetunisie.rns.tn/fr/prestations/programme-de-d%C3%A9veloppement-de-la-%C2%ABsant%C3%A9-num%C3%A9rique%C2%BB-en-tunisie*

39. **Lucas J.** Le point de vue des medecins. *Realites Familiales UNAF 2011;94:54-5.*

40. **Tunisian Society of Telemedicine & e-Health.** Telemedicine in Tunisia. *[En Ligne]. [Consulte le 15/07/2023], disponible a l'URL: https://www.telemedecine-tunisie.tn/content/la-t%C3%A9l%C3%A9m%C3%A9decine-en-tunisie*

41. **Khdimallah M.** e-sante en Tunisie: La telemedecine desormais legale. *La Presse, 06 March 2022.*

42. **Tobba.tn.** Teleconsultation medicale, Dossier Medical en ligne, Reseau Social medical & SanteLyna: espace de sante gratuit. *[Online]. [Consulte le 15/07/2023], disponible a l'URL: https://www.tobba.tn*

43. **Med.tn.** With Med, make an appointment online with your doctor otherwise. *[Online]. [Accessed 15/07/2023], available at URL: https://www.med.tn*

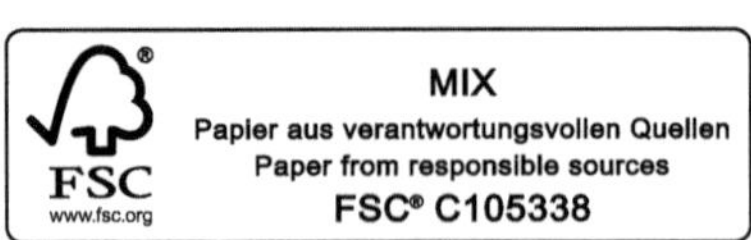

Printed by Books on Demand GmbH, Norderstedt / Germany